TO PEE *or* NOT TO PEE?

Advance Praise

"Shelia has created a simplistic yet empowering guide to bladder control. With over thirty years of experience as a physical therapist, certified Pilates instructor and fitness coach, she brings an integrated approach that every woman could benefit from for pelvic health and wellness."

— **Sonya Worthy Okolo**, Pelvic PT

"Shelia is an extremely knowledgeable physical therapist and demonstrates excellent skill as it relates to the areas of pelvic floor and lymphedema management. Shelia has over thirty years of experience as a physical therapist and has spent ten years specializing in the treatment of pelvic floor conditions. I've had the pleasure of working alongside and under the mentorship of Shelia. This proved to be an amazing experience as I was able to observe Shelia in action as she utilized a variety of techniques to help her patients improve their symptoms and reach their goals. During this time, I was able to glean from her expertise in the field which has proven to be of great benefit to the patient population that I serve. I am truly thankful for experiencing mentorship from one of the greatest in the field."

— **Tieya M. Qualls**, PT, DPT, PRPC

"*To Pee or Not to Pee* has extremely informative content regarding the female pelvic floor and pelvic health! I appreciated the diagrams, practical, factual and simplified details in this book, especially the kegel exercises. I've also had the pleasure of meeting Dr. Whiteman in person, and I want to emphasize that she genuinely cares for women's health, offering valuable insight that you can apply in your life immediately. I highly recommend Dr. Whiteman's book and program to other women who are experiencing leakage and to women like myself, who are focused on pelvic health in general. There's no need to wait until you have a problem, one can use this book for preventative health too!"

— **Josephine Grace**, Teacher, Author, Speaker

TO PEE
or NOT
TO PEE?

THE GUIDE FOR REDUCING AND
ELIMINATING URINARY INCONTINENCE

SHELIA CRAIG WHITEMAN
PT DPT CLT

NEW YORK

LONDON • NASHVILLE • MELBOURNE • VANCOUVER

TO PEE *or* NOT TO PEE?
THE GUIDE FOR REDUCING AND ELIMINATING URINARY INCONTINENCE

© 2021 **SHELIA CRAIG WHITEMAN** PT DPT CLT

Published in New York, New York, by Morgan James Publishing in partnership with Difference Press. Morgan James is a trademark of Morgan James, LLC. www.MorganJamesPublishing.com. Morgan James is a trademark of Morgan James, LLC. www.MorganJamesPublishing.com

ISBN 978-1-63195-074-2 paperback
ISBN 978-1-63195-075-9 eBook
ISBN 978-1-63195-076-6 audio
Library of Congress Control Number: 2020903731

Cover Design Concept:
Nakita Duncan

Cover Design:
Rachel Lopez
www.r2cdesign.com

Editor:
Nkechi Obi

Book Coaching:
The Author Incubator

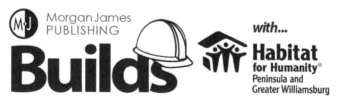

Morgan James is a proud partner of Habitat for Humanity Peninsula and Greater Williamsburg. Partners in building since 2006.

Get involved today! Visit
www.MorganJamesBuilds.com

To my wonderful husband and children who have given me the courage to keep learning, doing, and trying. I hope to make them as proud of me as I am of them. A special thank you to my fabulous daughter, Morgen A. Whiteman for the sketches contained in this book and her constant encouragement.

TABLE OF CONTENTS

....

CHAPTER 1

DID I JUST PEE ON MYSELF?

....

Who? Me?

H ave you ever had the "pleasure" of experiencing bladder leakage? I can remember the first time I waited way too long to get to a bathroom. When I started to pull down my pants, I felt a few drops of urine escape. My first thought was: *Did I just pee on myself?* Thankfully it did not become a regular occurrence, but it scared me enough to work to make sure it wouldn't.

Bladder leaks can affect anyone at any time. Although it is generally not a hot topic for discussion, many of us can relate to that feeling of a few drops of urine leaking out at some point in our lives. As a pelvic health physical therapist, I can say if you have experienced a leak or two, you are not alone. As a matter of fact, I would venture to say you have quite a bit of company. In the many years that I have focused on pelvic issues, incontinence, or bladder leaks, are one of the more common reasons people come to therapy for help. I frequently hear that if it wasn't for their physician's referral, the patient would not know that there is help available to stop leakage. Pelvic health physical therapy is becoming more common, making it much easier to find help to successfully stop or reduce bladder leakage.

Why Does It Take So Long to Get Help?

Several women I have worked with have a history of leakage going back years before I or any other therapist has seen them. Some of this may be due to just being so busy day after day. A small amount of leakage is very easy to ignore, especially if it is small enough to not change your daily activity. Many women are also in denial about what is going on. I have had women who wear a pantiliner every day think that they do not have leakage since a few small drops doesn't stop them from doing anything they want to do. I have heard that physicians are asking about bladder leaks during patient visits. Even my gynecologist has a questionnaire that asks if you are concerned or experienced leakage. This is progress! I hope this question becomes routine for all doctors to increase self-awareness. When leakage is treated early it is easier to stop.

You Are Not Alone

Amy is a fifty-year-old who complained of some bladder leakage whenever she had a cold. She told me the problem had been happening on and off for maybe five years or so. She has leaks when she coughs or sneezes. She is really only bothered at certain times of the year; she works with children and there is always one with a cold, runny nose, or cough. She thinks her leakage has been getting progressively worse, but this past year the leakage was really bad.

During our discussion, I asked her why she did not come for treatment when she first started leaking a few years ago. Her response: "I didn't look at it as a problem. Everyone has leakage at some point, right? Once I started using pantiliners, I really didn't consider it to be a problem. I am only here now because I am starting to leak through the pad. I don't want to have an accident."

If Amy acted at the beginning of her bladder problems, she could have started working on solving her problem early and may not have progressed to leaking an amount that was large enough to wet through her clothes. Better yet, she may have solved her problem sooner and with less effort. Isn't it interesting that we feel as long as something does not change our regular schedule or cause any issue, we can just deal with it and hope it goes away? Amy ignored seeking help for years because she could wear a pad and not change her daily routine. How many of you are doing the same thing? If this scenario feels familiar, I hope this book will help you to recognize and act to solve your problem.

Let's explore another example.

Berry is a forty-year-old IT professional with a busy and active social life. She works out at the gym three to four times a week and is in great shape. Almost every day when she gets to her apartment, the same exact thing happens. She puts her key in the door and immediately feels like she has to run to the bathroom! Sometimes she makes it, but sometimes she doesn't. She came to see me because the last few times—you guessed it—she didn't make it in time to avoid urinary leakage. Berry explained that this has been going on for years, but since she was always able to sprint to the bathroom in time, it was not a problem. After all, it had previously been only a few drops. However, once it went through her underwear onto her leg, it was something that she felt she could no longer ignore and sought help.

These are two very different, but typical, stories of how urinary incontinence can affect one's life. Take a moment and ask yourself if any of these situations sound familiar?

- Every time I turn around, I feel like I have to go to the bathroom.
- I can't get my work done. I feel like I just peed!
- I only leak a few drops when I cough or sneeze. It's no big deal.
- Women leak as they get older; that's just the way it is.
- I would like to go on a road trip with my friends, but what if I wet through my clothes? I can't take that chance. I don't think I will go this time.

There is help for bladder leaks and urinary incontinence. This book will help you understand what is going on and how it affects you. More importantly, it can give you information to help you to reduce and hopefully, eliminate your bladder leak. The first step though, is recognizing that the problem exists. If we can catch it early and work on it, then it is so much easier to get the result you want, which is to stop leakage for good.

There is no one set program for everyone that will effectively stop leakage. What you will learn in this book is how to identify what your problem is and how to start fixing it. Some of you may have already tried something that did not help or did not give you the results you wished for. It does take work and consistency to achieve your goals. What is the work? Keep reading—it is here in this book.

What Have You Tried to Fix Your Problem?

Have you been trying to do Kegels? Did it or is it working to help stop your leakage? How do you even know if you are doing them correctly? In my experience, the vast majority of the women I have treated were not even close to doing a correct Kegel.

Have you been only doing Kegels thinking that that is all you need to do? There are additional exercises and lifestyle changes you can try to help you become leak free. We can find the right combination of exercises and treatment to help you on your journey.

Effectively strengthening your pelvic floor muscles can sometimes be the missing link that is slowing your success in stopping your leakage. In a later chapter, you will learn the importance of mastering the proper way to perform a Kegel and other strengthening exercises.

Why Don't We Seek Help Sooner?

Do you have a little leakage that you are hoping will improve with time? Do you feel that you don't have the time right now to go to the doctor since it is just a few drops? After all, you don't leak all the time. Many women put off seeking help for years. As women we sometimes have many responsibilities and care for others first before taking care of ourselves. It is generally our nature to care for ourselves last. Please don't let this be you. If any of the examples or statements in this chapter resonate with you, take a minute and really note if you have the beginnings of this problem. I tell my patients, "Leakage is leakage." It can be a little, or it can be a lot. Does the amount change the fact that it is there? Just in case you are still not convinced, the answer is no!

Some of you have been really successful in ignoring the problem. This may be working out for you for now. Your bladder leaks might just be a minor inconvenience, and you might even think there is no problem. For some women, the problem may not even progress, it could just stay at a few drops only in certain situations. This could be where you stay. We just don't know. Let's look at this another way. What if you never had to worry that this might be the day you leak in public? What if you didn't have to spend money on pads or liners for protection. You can save that money and treat yourself to a new pair of shoes. I can't be the only shoe and purse lover here!

What if you can solve this problem early before it gets worse. Is that worth it? I hope you say, "yes." It would be wonderful if you did not wait years to seek answers to stop leakage. If you are using any type of pad, ask yourself is this just in case I leak a little? If so, then you just might be at the beginning of your leakage journey. Or maybe not, but it is worth investigating. Remember when it comes to urinary incontinence, we love the word *denial*. Just food for thought.

Bladder leaks can be embarrassing. Once it happens it is not something that can be easily forgotten. There will be that lingering fear of it happening again. Let's fix that!

Have you ever declined an invitation to a movie because you didn't feel confident you could sit through the entire movie comfortably? Let's fix that!

Are you missing out on living your life to the fullest because the fear of a bladder leak stops you from doing whatever it is you want to do? Let's fix that!

If we can solve your problem in the early stages, it is so much easier. The longer you wait the more work it takes to fix it.

Remember Amy and Berry from the beginning of this chapter? In both of these stories, they waited a long time—

actually years—before recognizing they had a leakage problem and then taking the next step of seeking help to stop leaking. This book will help you to understand normal bladder habits and what is not normal. This can help you to recognize sooner when it is time to seek help.

What Happens After You Seek Help?

Pelvic health therapists can treat more than incontinence or urinary leakage. There have been times when I have received a referral for a patient with abdominal pain or pain during intercourse. An initial visit includes an evaluation for the specific patient complaint and a screening for any other concerns or problems that may surface during the course of our discussion of her problem. Since bladder leaks are so common, they are part of the screening process. Many times the patient will report having to wear a pantiliner daily since she "may sometimes leak a few drops." Further questioning will reveal that she has had a few drops of leakage during stress activities—sneezing, coughing, or lifting—but did not think that there was anything that could be done about it, or even thought that this was a normal part of getting older. I sometimes feel that I have to almost convince them that a few drops are enough for concern and be considered bladder leakage. They honestly don't even realize that this could be true. Even though they were already wearing pads (for bladder leaks), they just did not associate the cause and effect.

Once they understand that bladder leaks usually do start out small and then progress to larger leaks, they are more than happy to begin the work to stop their leakage. This can usually be done in conjunction with whatever treatment is needed for their primary concern, i.e. their original reason for seeking help. They become more open to hearing and understanding that they do have leakage. Fortunately, they have found help for the problem that they were not aware they had.

If you are already seeking help for one problem and we discover your leakage as a related problem, you are in the right place for help. We can fix that, so let's go and do it.

I have noticed that for those women that are not seeking help for another issue, for example, pelvic pain, and their only problem is bladder leaks, it takes a longer time to seek help. By the time I see women in therapy for leakage, many times it has progressed so that the leak interferes in some way with their daily routine. Something changed and made them uncomfortable. Or, something made them unable to do something they wanted. You don't want to wait that long.

This book will help you understand what you can do to help stop or reduce bladder leaks. It is possible. Incontinence can be successfully reduced, but you have to understand and know what to do. I hope this first chapter has inspired you to start your journey to stop bladder leaks.

Are you tired of wishing the problem goes away? Let's work together and stop wishing and start acting.

We can do this.

You can do this.

Let's fix this!

CHAPTER 2

HOW I CAME TO SOLVE
THIS PROBLEM FOR OTHERS

···

I can still remember the day I decided I wanted to be a physical therapist. It was a long time ago, but some memories are so strong they are always suspended in time. Sometimes it feels like yesterday. I was still in high school and had a summer job at Children's Hospital in Buffalo, New York. I did odd jobs, mostly playing with the children that were hospitalized. By chance, I got to work, and really observe, in the physical therapy department. Watching the therapists work with these small children and help them get better inspired me. I decided then I wanted to be a physical therapist and never looked back.

Fun fact: I did pediatrics for about a year following graduation and decided children were not as fun as I thought.

Instead, my focus turned to working with adult orthopedics, neurology, and geriatrics, which I absolutely loved.

Over the next ten years I worked in many private settings and worked with a variety of different patients. I think I spent most of that time working in orthopedics, treating patients following surgery—hip and knee replacements, spinal surgeries and shoulder rotator cuff repairs with a few other ortho diagnoses thrown into the mix. One of the facilities where I worked was starting a program that focused on treating women following breast cancer, particularly the ones that developed lymphedema following medical intervention. This was the beginning of my transition to treating primarily women. I began to focus on physical therapy and oncology and became certified in lymphedema therapy and focusing on breast cancer rehabilitation. The outpatient clinic also started a women's health physical therapy program, and I began to take the classes and seminars to learn to treat this population. Between lymphedema and pelvic health, I found my niche as a physical therapist. These are my favorite groups to work with. When women with lymphedema or pelvic problems get relief from their symptoms, they are so grateful and happy. It is as if a weight has been lifted from their shoulders. I feel blessed to be a part of helping others live better and improve their quality of life. Eventually my patient base transitioned to primarily treating women with pelvic issues, but I do still on occasion have a breast cancer or lymphedema patient.

I do need to add that both lymphedema and pelvic health physical therapy require that the therapist do advanced training. Not every clinic has a pelvic therapist on staff, so please don't be afraid to ask your therapist what special training she has had and how long she has been working in the specialty. I was not the first therapist some of my patients had seen. Unfortunately, many of them had gone to therapy and did not see someone that specialized in the problem. The therapist was a physical therapist, though, and led the patient to believe she could help. Why would the patient think they could not? It is so important to ask just to make sure if you seek traditional physical therapy, you are being seen by the right person. There are more therapists who are getting the training, but it seems there still are not enough of us out there. If you choose in-clinic treatment, you have to have a therapist with additional training specific to pelvic health. It can be hard finding the right therapist with the actual training, but keep searching and get a good referral.

Once 90 percent of my patients were from pelvic health referrals, I really started having success. That is a lot of women over the years. Although I still love doing oncology and lymphedema, the need was just larger for great therapists with experience in the pelvic health field.

This is my story of becoming a pelvic health therapist. When you are blessed with the ability to help people find solutions and help with their problems and are successful doing it, I believe you are doing what you are meant to do.

How Can I Use This Book?

Did you know that when a therapist first starts on the journey to become a pelvic health therapist, the first condition she learns is how to treat incontinence? Why? It is because it is the easiest to learn and has a great success rate. I am not saying it does not take a lot of work to get results, but just think. Most of the time treatment is successful for those people who are committed. Once you come to the realization that you do have leakage, you have won half the battle.

After treating hundreds of women for leakage, I noticed that there are certain exercises and education that can help most women who just have urinary incontinence without other complications. If you have pelvic pain it may be a good idea to get an evaluation in person with a urogynecologist, urologist, or pelvic physical therapist to make sure there are no issues present that would need to be addressed before you can become successful in stopping your leakage.

I have used these same steps in this book to help many women including myself, with great results. Yes, I can get bladder leaks too if I get lazy and don't keep up with my exercises. Lucky for me, I know how to control it. One of the goals of this book is to outline that same program in easy to follow steps in the hope that you will have success to reduce your leakage as the other women I have worked with. I do believe the information in this book will lead you on the path of controlling your bladder leaks. Just imagine going out and not even thinking about the bathroom. What a pleasant dream that we can work on together to make a reality.

I don't want you to feel that you can't find help. If I wasn't a physical therapist, I think I would have a hard time trying to figure out where to go. This book came from the encouragement of my past patients. So many of them told me, "you should write a book." I finally listened and here it is. If any of you happen to pick up this book, thank you for your encouragement!

I believe that in order to get better, you need as much knowledge and information that would be helpful for you to understand what is happening. After all, it is your body, and you want to fix your problem. The patients I treated had such a high success rate because they learned the why, what, and how of their programs:

- Why is it important to know how my body works?
- Why should I do the program this way?

- What is the purpose of the exercises?
- How should I perform them?
- What is the proper way the program should be done?
- What do I need to do to get better?

Knowledge and understanding are the keys to your success. Yes, you can follow any program and maybe get better. But you want permanent results. If you don't understand the *why*, it is much more difficult to get long lasting results.

CHAPTER 3

HOW CAN THIS BOOK HELP ME?
AFTER ALL, IT IS ALL ABOUT YOU!

....

I am so pleased you decided to pick up this book to fix your leakage. Now, let's identify the best way to use this book so you will get the results you need.

One of the primary reasons that women feel they cannot solve this problem on their own is there is no direction on where to start. The most common advice most of us have gotten to stop leakage is to do Kegels. This is the main answer I get during evaluations when discussing what the patient has been trying to do on her own. I only wish that every time a woman was told to do a Kegel, she was also given real instructions on how to properly perform one. I think some women might have some success doing Kegels to stop their leakage, but it depends on catching it really early and the reason they started leaking in the first place. Unfortunately, the vast majority of women have not truly mastered the art of performing an effective pelvic floor contraction, aka Kegel. Therefore, they have not seen any success or enough success to do them long-term for effectiveness. If you have tried to do Kegels, did you know:

- What it is supposed to feel like when you are doing one?
- What muscle you are squeezing?
- What the purpose of doing them is?

During initial visits with me, patients would tell me that they did not really know how to know that they are doing Kegels the correct way. I would hear, "I was told to squeeze the muscles to try and stop the urine flow. That is all I have been trying to do."

Stopping bladder leaks is a lot more complicated than just squeezing your muscles and hoping for the best. Even if that suggestion were to help, how many times should you squeeze per day or per week? I can put that together for you so that there is a clear program you can try.

In later chapters, we are going to talk about the different types of leakage. Knowing which type is close to your symptoms will also give you a clearer picture of a program that will be effective for you. Many women do not receive the information that the program should be tailored to them. I can help you do that once you identify what your problem is. It would be great if stopping leaks was a one program fits all or as simple as squeezing and doing a Kegel. If that was the case, at least one third of the population would not have leakage. That number would be much, much lower.

We are going to identify the cause of most bladder leaks. Once you realize what is the most likely cause of your leakage, you can redirect your focus to being sure you are addressing it correctly. I would guess that over 80 percent of the women I have treated were unaware that improving this one factor would start them on the path to reducing symptoms.

How many of you know that, besides Kegels, there are other exercises that can be done to strengthen the pelvic area and help with leakage? In the treatment section of this book, you will learn additional exercises and activities you can perform to add to the chances of a successful outcome. By now, you may be wondering:

- How I can do this alone?
- Don't I need a health professional to help?
- Can I really do this?

The short answer is "yes." The long answer is the program we are going to be developing for you is very similar to what you would learn during our sessions. The difference is that I will be giving you the tools to help you decide on the most effective program to help instead of deciding for you. As you are reading through this book, some symptoms will be familiar, and they can go on your list to determine your program. Other signs and symptoms will not pertain to you, and that part of the program you don't have to do. It can seem complicated but really it is not. With this book you can also pace yourself a little more, but I want you to do the best you can and stay as consistent as you can once you decide to start working on this.

There are also some lifestyle changes you can try to help stop leakage. Solving this problem will take more than one approach to be effective and give you the results you wish for. There are a few ways to use this book effectively, and if you are working on your own, it can be a valuable resource to help you identify your type of bladder leak. If you are able to take your time and map out the plan that will help, you can find it here. The next step will be to have the determination to start and follow through with your plan to get the results you want and need.

Another way to use this book is as a reference. If you are currently working with a health professional for your leakage, this can perhaps give you more background to deepen your understanding of your program. I would like to take this opportunity to remind you that all therapists and health professionals do not treat the same way. What matters are the results. If you are working with your therapist and they have a different exercise, different repetition number, or different philosophy, please follow their guidance, especially if you are seeing improvement. If you have gone through a therapy program and notice some symptoms returning, this will be a great book for you to refresh your memory or try a few new techniques to get you back on track to keep your success going.

These are just a few suggestions of effective ways to use this book. The more understanding and knowledge you have regarding bladder leaks and urinary incontinence, the more empowered you will be to take control and work towards solving your problem. There are also some women that may have to work one-on-one with a therapist initially. Sometimes bladder leakage can be more complicated if there are other problems such as pain, muscle tightness, or trauma to the region. For more complex causes of bladder leaks you may need advanced treatment protocols. Should this be your case, this book can still provide an invaluable amount of background knowledge that can help in your treatment goals.

This book will help you:

- Identify your type of leakage.
- Know your basic anatomy.
- Effectively strengthen the right muscles.
- Do the right exercises.
- Add simple lifestyle changes to help reduce leakage.
- Reduce and/or stop your bladder leaks.

This is a great program for those women who have mild or light bladder leakage. If you leak a little, a lot, or even know you want to work on prevention of leakage in the future, let's continue on this journey to find your solution.

CHAPTER 4

HOW COMMON IS BLADDER LEAKAGE?

··

I t has been estimated that up to 50 percent of people have leakage in their lifetime. At any given time, a third of women have complaints about leaking during the day. You are not alone if this is your concern. As you can see, you have plenty of company. This is not a topic that is brought up regularly in conversation or you would know just how many friends and co-workers would be right with you on this topic. You know bladder leaks are a common problem when you see products for bladder leaks frequently advertised on television. These products would not be as available if there was no money to be made by promoting them.

As a pelvic health physical therapist, I talk about bladder leakage, or urinary incontinence (which is the term we use in the clinic), frequently. At social gatherings when the usual "What type of work do you do?" Q and A conversations start; I explain that I am a physical therapist who specializes in pelvic health problems. Most people don't have any idea what that means or that this specialty even exists. I explain that I help women with any pelvic issue that is going on between the belly button and upper thigh. For example, I can help with urinary leakage, pelvic pain and discomfort, and painful intercourse. Wow do those words open up a can of worms, as they used to say. Suddenly, I get a lot of, "Can I just ask you a quick question?" I don't mind at all; it is actually kind of fun. I love what I do. There are so many people affected by leakage, but they still are hesitant to talk about it even to their physicians. I get it; who wants to talk about urinary leaks? Not exactly an easy topic to bring up. It can be embarrassing to talk about something so personal. Fortunately, you have picked up this book and are taking the steps to understand what the heck is going on.

What Is Urinary Incontinence?

Urinary incontinence is most commonly referred to as bladder leaks. Same thing, same principle. Urinary incontinence just means that you leak urine and you cannot control it. Simple, right? However, there is always more to the story as we will find out in the later chapters. Did you know that there are different types of leakage and that the intervention may be different depending on the type? Before I started working in pelvic health, I had no idea. Granted that was around ten years ago when leakage was a secret no one wanted to talk about it. Even today with all the attention that has been given to leakage, many women (and men) stay in denial about the fact that they have actually had leakage for a long time! It is only after some years of dealing with the problem using pantiliners and other inventive means that they finally throw in the towel and ask for help.

Generally, once the leakage starts to change your lifestyle, you are ready to solve the problem and start to seek help. Sometimes the changes in lifestyle can be so gradual that you don't realize anything is different until you stop and think about it. For instance, have you noticed that:

- You know where every bathroom is in every store?
- You can't watch an entire movie without that uncomfortable "gotta go" feeling?
- You have missed parts of meetings/events because you had to go?
- You don't go to the gym to exercise for fear of leaks?
- You have leaked when you coughed or sneezed?

These are just a few examples of how leakage can start impacting one's lifestyle. Once bladder leaks stop your routine, or stops you from doing whatever you wish, it is time for a change.

In the following chapters, I will use different terms interchangeably. When you read them here or hear them on television or from your health professional, know that everyone is talking about the same thing. The terms used will depend on if we are speaking more clinically (urinary incontinence) or using the layman's term (leaks or bladder leakage).

Can This Happen to Me?

In the beginning of the chapter we identified that there is a 30 to 50 percent chance of having a bladder leak in your lifetime. That doesn't mean the full blown I have wet my pants scenario. Leakage can be just a few drops. Sometimes, leaks are temporary, perhaps due to illness, urinary tract infection or medication. Other times, leaks can happen for an extended period commonly due to pelvic floor muscle weakness. In the later chapters, it should become clearer whether your leakage is temporary or whether it is time for you to seek help.

Let's go back for a minute and recap the information presented so far. I have found that recaps and reinforcements of information given at each step helps understanding.

Better understanding leads to better outcomes.

So far, we've established that:

- Bladder leakage is very common.
- Bladder leakage and urinary incontinence can mean the same thing.
- We don't like to talk about it but that doesn't make it go away.
- It can be temporary due to illness or medication.
- Leakage can be a few drops or enough to run down your leg. If you didn't want it to happen, it is considered urinary incontinence. It can be long-standing, in which case help is needed.

The Urinary System

I have used the words "bladder leak" several times already in this book, but what does the bladder do? Let's take a short, and I mean very short, review of the urinary system.

Diagram 1: Frontal view of the Female Urinary Tract System

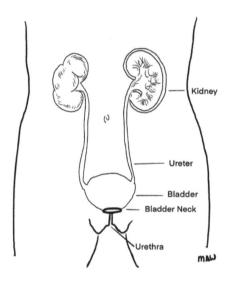

Let's look **Diagram 1** from top to the bottom to better understand the urinary system.

Kidneys

These two organs work all day to constantly filter the waste from your blood and produce about thirty-two to sixty-four ounces of urine daily.

Ureters

Thin tubes that carry the urine to the bladder.

Bladder

A balloon-shaped organ that holds the urine until you are ready to go to the bathroom. It can hold up to *two cups of urine*—around 16 ounces—before you really have to go. The bladder has a muscle layer that expands or stretches as it fills. When it is filled to capacity, the bladder sends a signal to the brain that it is time to empty. The bladder contracts to send the urine out of the body

Urine is constantly dripping into the bladder; it doesn't flow in rapidly, or in large quantities. It is just a steady drip that can be fast or slow depending on your hydration level.

Urethra

A tube that goes from the bladder to the outside to get rid of the urine.

This is the first, basic lesson that will help you identify the anatomy we will refer to throughout some of the book.

What Are Normal Bladder Habits?

The average bladder can hold about fourteen to sixteen ounces of urine before you get that strong urge that it is time to go. At that time, the bladder has expanded and stretched. Once the bladder stretches to a certain point, it will send a signal to the brain that it is time to empty. There is a very strong connection between the brain and bladder. This connection is very important when we are working towards staying dry. Sometimes the focus is on retraining and changing some of the bad habits that have been created when leakage has been present for a while. Generally, the brain-bladder connection works like this: the bladder sends a signal to the brain that it feels full and it is time to empty. The brain then sends a signal to the muscles of the bladder to relax and to let the urine flow out. Normally you should be going to the bathroom six to eight times per day. If you are older, it may be one or two times more but, still, no more than every two hours.

When you do urinate, the flow should be steady, and you should not have to push. Urine should flow out easily. The sphincter muscles of the pelvic floor at bottom of the ureter relaxes, opening so urine should be able to easily flow out. You should take your time. Make sure you are not rushing. You want to make sure you completely empty the bladder. Trying to hurry and speed up the process may backfire. If you are not able to completely empty because you are rushing the process, guess what? There will still be urine in the bladder taking up space. Remember, your bladder can only hold sixteen ounces comfortably. Since the bladder is constantly filling, it may not take as long for the bladder to refill since it already has a larger residual volume from incomplete emptying. If you recall, there is normally a two-and-half to three hour wait between voids, but if it is already say, a third of the way full, it will take a shorter amount of time to fill, and you may need to go to the bathroom sooner.

Let's look at it a different way. Say you left five ounces in the bladder because you were in a hurry and could not take the extra few minutes to wait until your bladder was almost empty. If your bladder can hold sixteen ounces (and some can hold more or less—that is the average), you are starting already with five ounces still in the bladder. It will take less time for you to feel the urge to go again since you only have room for eleven more. I know that is a lot of math! Bottom line: take your time so you won't have to go to the bathroom as often.

If you are staying hydrated, it is normal to go to the toilet every three to four hours to pee. Going past four hours can mean you aren't drinking enough water, or you are ignoring the urge to go, which is a bad idea. Remember, that urge is your bladder signaling to the brain that it is filling up and to be on alert to open that sphincter muscle. It doesn't necessarily mean that it is time to go. You can get a small urge signal that the bladder is filling but not enough that you have to go to the bathroom, or you can get an urgent signal. When the big urge comes, it is time to go unless you are retraining your brain for frequency which we will discuss later.

Think about this, every time you get the urge, you do not want to go and empty. If you did, you would be in the bathroom every hour, and who has time for that? Besides, that is not the way our bodies work anyway. We just learned that information earlier. Here is the takeaway about urge. Because you have an urge does not mean you have to jump up and go to the bathroom. What it means is that your brain-bladder connection is working the way it should. Please, though, don't ignore the urge, especially if it is strong and you haven't gone to the bathroom in over four hours. That can cause another issue or make you more likely to leak just because your bladder is full.

Remember, urine constantly drips into the bladder and it has a capacity. You want to try not to have over-filling become a habit. On the other hand, you want to also try to avoid going to the bathroom just in case. What this means is going to the bathroom before an activity just in case you have the urge when it may be inconvenient. Let me give you an example. I just went to the bathroom about thirty minutes ago and decided I am going to go sit outside for a bit and read. Should I go to the bathroom again right before I go outside so I won't have to come back in? What do you think? Better yet, how many of us have done this just so be on the safe side? I hope your answer is no, I shouldn't go because I just went. That brain-bladder connection is pretty consistent. You don't want to train the bladder to think it is okay to empty frequently, or it will be an unwelcome habit you will have to work to break. Who wants to have to go to the bathroom every hour? Not me.

What Are Good Bladder Habits?

One of the most important things you can do to maintain good bladder health is to stay hydrated. The recommended amount of fluid intake varies depending on what information sources you are using, but I still go by the standard of at least six to eight, eight-ounce cups of liquid daily. Of course, if your doctor tells you otherwise, use that recommendation. If you are not hydrated enough, your urine can become more concentrated which can be irritating to the bladder.

Let's take a quick urinary tract review.

In Diagram 1, the parts of the urinary system were identified. The function of the **kidney** is to filter waste from the blood. The tubes that move the urine from the kidneys to the bladder are called the **ureters**. The **bladder** holds urine until it can be eliminated through the **urethra**.

It is extremely important to stay well hydrated for good bladder health. When you don't drink enough liquids, urine can have a higher concentration of waste products. Concentrated urine is irritating to the bladder and your body tries to remove it as soon as possible. Instead of being able to wait three to four hours between voids we now know should be the normal interval, it could be as little as one to two hours because your body is trying to rid itself of the more concentrated urine that is irritating the bladder lining. This can lead to frequency, or having to go to the bathroom too often, which can be just as embarrassing as leakage.

You now have a basic understanding of the importance of the urinary system, what it does, and how to keep it doing what it is supposed to do. Let's continue to explore some additional background information so you will be prepared to solve your problem.

CHAPTER 5

ONCE YOU UNDERSTAND THE BASICS, IT ISN'T SO HARD

....

I n the previous chapter, you have already had your first anatomy lesson when you learned how the urinary system works. Now, it is time to get a little deeper understanding of the pelvic area so that when you learn the steps in this program, you will fully understand why a particular exercise or movement is important. Let's start by learning what is in the pelvis and where these parts are located and positioned in relation to each other.

Cross Section of the Female Pelvis

The sketch on the next page shows a cross section of a female pelvic region. The main organs of the pelvic floor are the bladder, uterus, and rectum. You can see where they are in relation to each other. The pelvic floor muscles are located

Diagram 2: Cross Section of the Pelvis

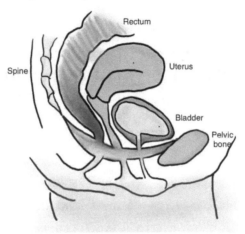

at the bottom or low part of the pelvis. These muscles start at the pubic (pelvic) bone in the front of the body to the coccyx or tailbone at the back. Think of these muscles like a sling or hammock that help to support all of the structures and organs in the area. The pelvic floor has several layers of muscles and connective tissue that are located at the bottom of the pelvis or the hip area.

Diagram 3: Muscle Layers 1 and 2

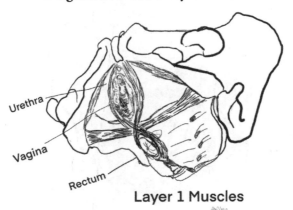

Urethra

Vagina

Rectum

Layer 1 Muscles

Where and What is the Pelvic Floor?

There are three layers of muscle that form the pelvic floor. The surface has layers 1 and 2.

The function of the first layer is to help support the vagina, rectum, and urethra. The first layer also aids in supporting arousal and orgasm in both women and men.

The second layer contains the sphincter muscles. These are the muscles that close off the openings, keeping them closed when you don't want to urinate or have a bowel movement. They also are able to relax when it is time to open to allow the release of urine and bowel contents.

Diagram 4: Pelvic Muscle Layer 3

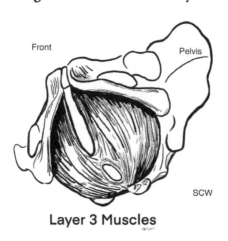

Layer 3 Muscles

Layer 3

The primary function of the third layer of muscles is support. These muscles are always working to support the organs in the pelvis. They especially keep the bladder, uterus, and rectum in place. This very important third layer works with your abdominal muscles to provide stability to the lower part of your trunk.

The pelvic floor is extremely important to keep everything where it should be. Many people do not know that the pelvic floor consists of three different muscle layers, each layer having a different function. Knowing your anatomy will help you to visualize and understand which muscles need to be strengthened so you can perform a proper Kegel exercise or pelvic floor muscle contraction. It will help you learn why just squeezing may not be enough to be sure your pelvic floor muscles are properly contracting and being strengthened. When we think about a typical Kegel, it is described as more of a squeeze. Doing just a squeeze may not even reach the third layer, which you have just learned has the primary job of keeping everything where it is supposed to be. In order for you to stay dry and control leakage, each one of these layers becomes very important and has either a structural, support, or control job in keeping you dry.

Let's review the pelvic floor muscle layers:

Layer 1 provides support for the canals that open to the outside of the body; the vagina, urethra and rectum.

Layer 2 contains the sphincter muscles that control when you urinate or have a bowel movement. When contracted, you remain continent i.e. you do not leak. When these muscles relax, the urethra or rectum can open to allow you to urinate or have a bowel movement.

Related but unrelated side note: because bowel is a solid, the rectal sphincter is usually stronger. Because of the way the muscle fibers run, there will be overflow movement around the vagina if you squeeze the rectum, meaning with a strong rectal squeeze you will naturally feel some contraction around the vaginal canal. Many women with poor muscle strength are able to compensate for pelvic floor muscle weakness this way. Doing a good, strong rectal sphincter contraction can feel like you are doing a great Kegel. This is another reason why instruction on how to do a proper Kegel or pelvic floor muscle contraction is so helpful. There are other muscles other than those of the pelvic floor that can make it feel as if you are strengthening correctly. Unfortunately, if your strengthening exercise is not hitting all the muscle layers or you are only contracting the surface layers but not the deeper third layer, it may be hard to get the results that you want, which is to be dry all the time.

Layer 3 is the muscle hammock the keeps everything in its place. This layer must be strengthened for long-term success from urinary and bowel incontinence primarily by reducing the incidence of pelvic organ prolapse (POP).

Test Your Knowledge Checkpoint 1

In which layer do you find the muscles that close off the urethra and the rectum to prevent leaks from bladder and bowel?

If you said layer 2, you are absolutely correct!

This does not mean that the other two layers are unimportant. All three layers of pelvic muscles must work to help keep you dry. They all work together very closely. If one layer is not working properly, the other muscle layers are not able to work at their peak level. This is why when I am teaching techniques to stop leakage, I want you to focus on the entire pelvic floor and not just one part. If all parts are not working optimally, then you won't get the desired long-lasting result.

Why is stopping leakage so hard? We just learned that it is not a simple matter of squeezing the pelvic muscles or whatever one might feel they are tightening down there. It has to be done correctly, and you need to target the right muscles. Is it becoming clearer why a deeper understanding of what needs to be done is needed for success?

Without background knowledge, how would anyone who has not taken anatomy know there are three muscle layers and that they do more than one thing?

If you need to return to this chapter as we move through to identify your type of leakage and your program, please do come back as many times as you need to remember. Especially review the diagrams to help remember where things are. Once you understand the basics, you can see why this is not a one-squeeze-fits-all problem. On the flip side; once you understand the basics, it is easier to figure out what you need to stop your problem.

CHAPTER 6

WHAT TYPE OF
LEAKAGE DO I HAVE?

....

Wouldn't it be so easy if there was one type of leakage and everyone could do the same program and get great results? That would be my wish for all of us but, alas, it is not meant to be. Let's talk about the main types of urinary incontinence and a few very related problems. You might have symptoms of one, two, or all of the types. Not to worry, though, even if you think each and every one is your story; they all have a solution. Let's look at a few examples of what leakage may look like.

Stress Urinary Incontinence

A.W. came to therapy very frustrated and unhappy. She is in her mid-50s and recently had a really bad cold. She noticed that every time she coughed or sneezed, she leaked urine. Most of the time it was just a few drops, so she was okay with that. But then she began to notice that when she coughed, more than a few drops came out. She immediately saw her doctor who referred her to pelvic physical therapy. She reported that although her cold was mostly gone, the leakage had remained, and it seemed like it was not getting any better. The leaking began when her cold was really bad.

"I just went and got some pantiliners thinking that once the cold was gone and the coughing and sneezing was better, I would be fine. It has been three months, but I still notice that if I sneeze, I am still leaking. What is going on here? I am too young to start leaking all the time," she said.

W.E. is an active woman in her 40s who is in the armed forces. Apparently, there are yearly fitness tests that they have to pass, which include running and push-ups. She came to me because she started to leak a lot when she started practicing for her yearly exam. She noticed leaking while running and also while doing her push-ups. She was starting to panic. It was coming up soon, and all she wanted to do was to stop the leaking enough to get past the tests for the year.

These are classic stories of stress urinary incontinence (UI). Stress urinary incontinence is leaking with increased intra-abdominal pressure and/or physical activity. A person will usually complain of leakage during an activity that requires a short burst of energy or pressure as in the case of a cough or sneeze. It can occur when you cough, sneeze, or exercise. It can also occur when lifting a heavy object. It usually starts with a few drops but can progress to being enough to wet through your clothing. As time goes on, if it is not addressed, it can get worse.

Stress UI can occur at any age. I have had patients in their 20s as well as in their 80s with stress UI.

Urge Urinary Incontinence

B.T. came to therapy very frustrated and afraid. She was in a meeting and needed to go to the bathroom, but the time just was not right. She could not get up in the middle of a presentation to run to the bathroom and back. So, she stayed, uncomfortably. She told me she couldn't even focus on the presentation much less remember what they were even talking about. At the end of the meeting, she managed to sprint to the bathroom, but it was a little too late to avoid really wetting through her underwear and the small pantiliner she always wore. She stated that she had been having leakage for years but that so far, she had never leaked through her clothes.

V.C. has been having little problems with leakage for years. She is in her early 60s and has a very busy life. She has been dealing with her problem by wearing pantiliners, just in case, and changing them as needed. To her, a little leakage was just a small annoyance that she did not think was important enough to have to stop and take care of it. Time just kept going until she honestly couldn't even tell me when the problem started; it seemed so long ago. As the story goes, her problem was getting worse, but it usually takes a big event to command the attention needed to work on this problem.

V.C. came home from work last week, put her key in to unlock her door, and felt a strong urge to get to the bathroom. Well, she didn't make it, and it ran down her leg. It was enough to convince her that now was the time to find help. This is urge urinary incontinence. Other common triggers for urge UI are:

- Pulling down your pants to go to the bathroom.
- Putting your key in the lock to get into your home.
- The sound of running water.

Urge incontinence (UI) is uncontrolled leakage of large amounts of urine when you least expect it. This is one of the more frustrating types of leakage. You don't know when it is going to happen or how much leakage will occur. It can be enough to actually wet through your clothes and be noticeable. I can't tell you, though, how many women wait until it gets to the wetting through your clothes phase before they seek help. Although leakage is a serious problem, many times it starts slowly and is just a small inconvenience that a little pantiliner can hide. Actually, in my experience, most women do not even try to find help until the problem changes something that is a part of their routine and they can no longer do it, or the leakage is just so pronounced that it can no longer be ignored. Some of its characteristics include:

- Leaking urine when you don't expect it.
- Leaking that can be large amounts.

Mixed Urinary Incontinence

V.A. came to her evaluation worried because she was leaking all the time. She had progressed to using adult diapers so that she would feel secure during the day and not worry about leaks. She was worried that people would know she had leakage because they could see the diaper or even smell urine if they came close enough. It seemed as if *everything* caused her to leak. She reported leaking during cough/sneeze/exercise. She reported leaking after having a sudden urge to urinate or hearing water running.

What V.A. was experiencing was Mixed Urinary Incontinence, which usually refers to having symptoms of both stress and urge urinary incontinence. Since she has symptoms of more than one type of leakage, she would benefit from doing the exercises included in both programs to target the correct muscles. V. A. has just a little more work to do to help her leakage but since some exercises can be combined, she can still expect to see improvement in her symptoms.

Overactive Bladder

S.C. story is just a little different. She was frustrated and unhappy. She felt as if half of her day was spent either in the bathroom or looking for one. She had the urge to go all the time even if she just went thirty minutes ago. She did not feel comfortable going to the movies because she couldn't sit that long. The same thing went for church. Going out with friends was becoming a nightmare because she was the one who always had to stop and go.

There are similar stories, but do you ask yourself:

- Do I feel as if I need to go to the bathroom all the time?
- Am I already wearing or tempted to buy incontinence pads or the really pretty incontinence underwear that I see on television?

This could be overactive bladder or OA.

Symptoms of OA are usually a combination of frequency and urgency. With this type of incontinence, you feel like you have to go to the bathroom all the time even if you just went. In chapter 4, we discussed good bladder habits. One of them was going to the bathroom every three to four hours. That is a happy and healthy bladder. With overactive bladder, you will feel the urge to go urinate even fifteen minutes after you have just used the bathroom. This can be frustrating. The other part of OA is you go to the bathroom more than every two to two and a half hours. This is frequency.

Remember that strong brain-bladder connection? Your bladder is sending a signal to the brain that it is time to go (urge), and your brain does what it is supposed to do which is relax those muscles so that the urine is released. Urge is just a signal that it *might* be time to empty, but it doesn't mean that you have to empty. We will learn more about when urge should be acted on or ignored in a following chapter.

Frequency is another issue we can solve with a good retraining program. Frequency is interesting because it actually can be a stand-alone problem. During the training to treat incontinence, we practice some information that we will use on ourselves. In the class, we learned about normal bladder habits, and we all had to fill out a two-day bladder diary (we will talk about them later) to see if any of us had symptoms. The instructor even made a bet that most of us would find something that could be considered not normal. Turns out she was right. Many of us in class found out that we did have a habit that we could improve. My diary showed that I was going to the bathroom every one and a half hours from the time I got up until early afternoon. I had frequency! Needless to say, I spent the next few weeks working on this to get back to a comfortable three to four-hour wait.

When we get to the treatment section in a later chapter, we'll talk about how you can find out if you have frequency or the beginning of the problem. I had it and didn't even know it. Luckily, I hadn't reached the "I can't sit though class" stage yet. I was able to fix my problem early before it changed my daily patterns so much that it was disruptive.

To recap, frequency is just as it sounds—you go to the bathroom too frequently. Similarly, urgency simply means you feel as if you need to pee urgently. There are no true triggers and they can come with a little or a lot of leakage.

Nocturia (Knock-tur-e-a)? Knock What?

D.K. came to me unable sleep at night because she was up going to the bathroom every few hours. She stated she would go to bed at 11 p.m. and wake up like clockwork at 1:30, 3:30 and finally 5:00 a.m. She had to get up for work at 6:00 a.m. She was just exhausted and wanted to know what could be done. This had been going on for years but had gotten progressively worse so that it happens: Every. Single. Night.

This is an example of Nocturia. No, I am not making this up. There is a name for everything! Nocturia can be either having the urge to go to the bathroom several times per night and successfully running to the toilet or, unfortunately, either wetting the bed or leaking on the way to the bathroom. None of those scenarios are a good thing, agreed?

Post Pregnancy Leakage

V.P. had a beautiful baby boy about fifteen months ago. There were no complications during the pregnancy. Her adorable bundle of joy weighed 8.5 pounds at birth. V.P. had some leakage during the pregnancy; however, her doctor assured her that this was common, so she wasn't really worried at that time.

She finally let her doctor know during a routine visit that she had never stopped leaking since her pregnancy and was sent to see me. She primarily complained of leaking throughout the day. There were no real triggers except she noticed more leakage when she picked her son up or tried to exercise.

This is a typical story of post-pregnancy leakage that did not stop following birth. It is normal for a woman to have leakage during pregnancy and shortly after a vaginal birth. During pregnancy, the baby is growing, and the uterus is expanding, muscles, and ligaments are stretching and there is increasing weight in the pelvic region. Generally, though, as a woman heals following birth, many of these symptoms disappear as her body begins to return to normal. There is a small group of women that need a little more help to get back to normal.

This is an example of someone with continued problems with leakage following childbirth. The takeaway from this story is: leakage during pregnancy happens. But if it is still happening months after delivery, think about seeking some extra help in order to fix this. There is help for you.

There is one other thing I wonder if you picked up on in the post-pregnancy story. She had increased leakage when she picked her son up. What type of leakage could that be? Remember you can have more than one type of leakage at a time. If you said stress urinary incontinence you get a gold star! Great catch!

Now that you understand what type of leakage you have; we can begin to formulate your program!

CHAPTER 7

WHERE DO I START?

....

We learned that there are different types of incontinence that may be accompanied by frequency. To review, we discussed:

- Stress Urinary Incontinence
- Urge Urinary Incontinence
- Mixed Urinary Incontinence
- Overactive Bladder
- Nocturia

It is time to think about where your symptoms fit into one or more of these descriptions. This is the first step in beginning to find the program that can help you.

Identify Your Type

In the previous chapter, I talked about the class that I attended and having to fill out the two-day bladder diary. Bladder—and sometimes bowel—diaries are very effective. Basically, you track when you go to the bathroom over either a two or three-day period. It sounds difficult, but it really isn't unless you are always going to the bathroom and have a lot of leakage. If that is the case, then doing a bladder diary will definitely help you to learn what your good and bad habits are. This information can really be an eye opener. Remember how I found urinary frequency when I did my diary? Well, another thing I found out is that one of the nights I had nocturia. Using some of the exercises you will learn about, I was able to normalize these symptoms.

Now let's use a bladder diary to help identify your symptoms. A bladder diary can help you to determine if there are any triggers that contribute to your leaks or if you go to the bathroom too frequently during the day. The bladder diary can also give you a wealth of information about your bladder habits. It is easy to make a chart for yourself. There are many examples on the Internet, or if you contact me, I can send you one to use. At a minimum, you want your bladder diary to include the following information:

- The time of day
- The amount of water you drink (quantity and time)
- The times you eat
- The time and frequency of bathroom trips over a 24-hour period including nighttime voids
- How badly you had to go
- How much leakage you had

Once you have this information, you can look for patterns or triggers as to why there may be leakage and/or frequency. If you are serious about stopping or reducing your leakage, I would recommend doing a bladder diary for a minimum of two days. I generally have women do a three-day diary, two weekdays and a weekend, since many of us have different patterns of activities between weekdays and the weekend.

Interpreting Your Bladder Diary

Once you have done a two or three-day diary, you'll want to look at the results for patterns. Let's say you notice you go to the bathroom every one and a half to two hours in the morning like I did. We learned the normal time between voids is three to four hours, so you may have frequency because you went to the bathroom too frequently in a short time period.

This can also tell you if longer than four hours passes between each time you go. That is not a situation we address in this book, but it could be a sign of poor hydration or urinary retention. If you think you have signs of urinary retention, please make an appointment to discuss treatment options with a physician.

Your diary can let us know if there are any foods that irritate your bladder and cause frequency. We can see if there is any leakage throughout the day and what might be a possible trigger. We can note whether or not there are frequent trips to the bathroom at night. I love bladder diaries! They are a simple tool, which may be a little tedious to fill out, but the information they give is invaluable. Once it is completed, you will now have the information to begin identifying your symptoms.

Now, let's explore some additional information you can find from looking at your diary. You are looking for patterns. Do you go too frequently? What are your triggers? Do you get up frequently at night? Look at your pattern and see if it reinforces your initial idea of the type of leakage you have. Does it fall into the same category as before?

- Stress UI
- Urge UI
- Mixed UI

- Overactive
- Nocturia

Test Your Knowledge Checkpoint 2

The questions below will test your understanding of the types of urinary incontinence. You can find the answers below.

Question	Answer
1. Jane notices that she has a few drops of leakage when she coughs. This is:	
2. Mary finds that her trigger for leaks is hearing running water. This is:	
3. A.J. sees a pattern of going to the bathroom every hour but only in the morning. This is:	
4. S.C. noticed that she did not go to the bathroom all morning; this was a period of over four hours. This is:	

5. Sue sees that she is leaking all the time, but she can't find a pattern. This is:

6. Ethel notices she is getting up two to three times per night to go to the bathroom. This is:

Bladder Diary Answers

1. This is stress urinary incontinence (UI). Stress UI is triggered by any sudden movements that increase intra-abdominal pressure such as a sneeze, cough, or lifting a heavy object without bracing and using proper breath patterns.

2. Having a strong urge to urinate while hearing running water is a sign of urge UI. Triggers can include, the sound of running water, unlocking a door to get into the house, or pulling down your underwear to use the bathroom.

3. This problem is just as you would expect. This is an example of frequency. She is going to the bathroom too often during the morning. Unless she is drinking very large quantities of water, she should still be able to hold a pattern of every three to four hours.

4. You would get number four right only if you were paying close attention! This is the opposite of frequency. It is Urinary Retention. Although we are not going to talk about it in this book, this also is not normal and should be discussed with your physician or appropriate health professional.

5. The dreaded all the time leakage. There can be several reasons this happens. If you said mixed UI, I will give you an A. It just seems like there is leakage if you cough, sneeze, walk, stand up, exercise or just about anything. Mixed UI can be reduced or eliminated; it just may take a little more time and effort.

6. Here is the last one. Who has heard of nocturia prior to reading this book? If you are getting up several times to go to the bathroom, with or without leakage, you have nocturia.

So how did you do? Using a simple bladder diary can give so much information to help you to identify your problem. If keeping a three-day bladder diary is not your thing or you just don't want to do it, you can figure out your problem by looking at your symptoms. You will still get a good idea of what is going on, but you could miss a pattern that if acted upon could improve your outcome. The bladder diary is great because many women have more than one problem or concern. If you do the diary correctly, you can sometimes identify the other problems that are not as bothersome so they are not missed.

Kegels Explained

There are several different types of urinary incontinence and bladder leakage problems. There is one thing though that is common for over 90 percent of women with this problem: poor pelvic floor muscle strength. If women could master how to do an effective Kegel and stay consistent with the exercise, I believe half of their leakage complaints would be solved.

The Kegel exercise primarily targets the pelvic floor muscles. In therapy, we don't just test your pelvic muscle strength by seeing how hard you can squeeze the muscle. Let me first explain that if you have ever gone or plan to go to therapy for incontinence, it is a very intimate experience. The most accurate way to determine your strength is by using a gloved finger inserted into your vagina since we can feel and palpate all of the muscles there. That is especially the most accurate way to get to the layer 3 muscles. Remember, those are your hammock support muscles, so they are all the way at the top of your vagina and very easy to find if you have a skilled therapist.

When I am doing the assessment, I look for a few things that will give me an idea of why this has happened. I focus on the strength or the lack thereof. In assessing strength, I am looking for:

- How hard you can squeeze my finger
- Whether or not I can feel a lift like you are pulling my finger up when you squeeze
- If you can hold the contraction for up to ten seconds without fail
- If you can do fast contractions and release in a coordinated manner
- If you can release your contraction quickly or if it is difficult for you to relax

Each of these are important to reduce leakage.

It is very important to be able to fully relax the pelvic floor muscles in order to do an effective Kegel and improve your coordination to help your control. Practice abdominal breathing first with a focus on just letting your pelvic muscles relax as you exhale. This is not an active push of the muscle. Passively relax and let go of your pelvic floor muscles. Don't skip over this step! It is just as important as learning how to effectively strengthen these muscles. If you are unable to relax your pelvic muscles, it is difficult to get a strong contraction. If your muscles are hypertonic or tight you must learn how to relax them before you can progress to the strengthening step.

Let's take some time and work on doing a good Kegel. In the beginning, I really want you to practice lying down so that you can get a good base and better strength before you go to gravity dependent positions of sitting or standing. Lie on your back on a bed with your legs supported on pillows or a wedge (hook-lying). Start with abdominal breathing to relax the pelvic floor. Place one hand above your belly button. This is so you can feel if you are using your abdominal muscles to help you. You can place the other hand on your thigh or glute muscles. Both are common muscles used to substitute for a weak pelvic floor.

Close your eyes. When you begin to squeeze the muscles of the pelvic floor, I want you to also think about lifting them up towards your stomach. Another good visualization is to think of your pelvic floor as an elevator. Start your contraction from the bottom, squeeze *and lift* the contraction up to the top floor (as high as you can).

This takes practice and time to master. If you can feel a strong lift without using substitute muscles, you have it. Make sure though you are not performing any of the common substitutions:

- Squeezing your glutes
- Holding your breath
- Pulling in your belly button
- Squeezing your inner thighs together

I know it is a lot! This is why people don't do as well as they could, your foundation for strengthening has to be good. You need to understand that the squeeze must be combined with a lift in order to be effective. After you understand and are able to do a good Kegel, you are on the way to improving your problem. Take your time on this part. In the clinic, sometimes it takes weeks to master it. It is okay; your pelvic floor weakness did not happen overnight, and it will not be solved overnight.

You can even stop reading right here until you can do a Kegel. This is an important step no matter which type of leakage you have identified as the problem. I want you to be able to do a good contraction that includes a lift before you add anything else to the program. We are setting the stage for success not failure. Strengthening your pelvic floor muscles is one of the main keys to success. Learning how to do the exercise that actually will strengthen these muscles is time well spent. The programs to reduce and eliminate leakage are based on the proper execution of a Kegel. Once you understand how to do one and can feel the muscles actually lifting, you can add onto your program.

Although mastering Kegels are a vital step to reducing leakage, they are just one part of the program. There are a few more things you can do to make sure you are successful. Once you are confident you are doing the exercise correctly it is time to move on to the next chapter to continue the work!

CHAPTER 8
LET'S START THE PROGRAM

....

Step 1: You have Identified Your Problem

Once you have identified your symptoms and problem, you have taken a major step in fixing it. If you did a bladder diary for two or three days, you may have even noticed you have more than one concern regarding not so good bladder habits. This is not really a cause for concern. When reviewing the information from your diary or reviewing your symptoms, there are usually other issues. I see this most of the time in the clinic while gathering the information to begin treatment. Luckily, with this program, you will be able to address several problems at once, since they are generally interrelated. An example would be that you notice stress UI and frequency. You will be able to add suggestions from both programs to solve both of these issues.

You have already identified the triggers and kind of leakage you are experiencing. So now, you also are going to learn how to control urinary frequency and nocturia.

Step 2: Strengthening

Most, if not all, women will benefit from starting with a strengthening program. We ended the last chapter discussing Kegels and their importance in strengthening the muscles of the pelvic floor. Before you begin Step 2, it is important that you have practiced doing a Kegel. Depending on the length of time since you have done one or if you ever have, this may be the most difficult part of your journey. Initially, the contraction does not have to be perfect by any means, but it is important that you begin to build on a foundation of doing it correctly.

One of the hardest things is to retrain someone on how to do a proper Kegel. Once your brain has accepted a certain way of doing something and you have to change that way of doing it, it becomes a retraining process. The only requirement is to feel the beginnings of a squeeze. You don't have to worry about closing anything just yet, and I certainly don't expect you to be able to feel that lift of the muscles at this point.

If you are at the point that you have perfected the contraction and lift, congratulations! That is a large part of mastering Step 2. If you are still struggling with knowing if you are even moving any muscle, try to use a mirror and see if you can see movement while you are doing a Kegel. Lie or sit down and aim the mirror towards your vagina. You should see a close and lift at your vaginal opening. Even if you only see a small movement, as long as you are isolating that area, you are right on track. Refer back to the substitutions that you want to avoid to strengthen the right muscles. If you need to keep practicing using a mirror until you are confident that you are on the right track, that is fine. It will help you to be sure you are targeting the correct muscles.

If this is all very new to you and you just learned there is such a thing as a pelvic floor, don't worry if it takes you a little longer to feel the squeeze and lift. It will take time especially for the lift. Be persistent and practice a few contractions daily— with persistence you can learn how to do them.

I do want you to remember the no's for Kegels. These are very important:

- No holding your breath
- No squeezing your inner thighs together
- No strong pulling in your belly button
- No clenching or squeezing your glutes (butt)

There is one more that may be the most important:

- *No pushing the muscles out or bearing down*

Think only *lift*!

The Stress Urinary Incontinence Strengthening Program

As you will recall from earlier chapters, Stress UI is leakage during activities or situations when there is a sudden, quick change in abdominal and pelvic floor pressure. This is your sneeze, cough, or lifting something heavy and then feeling either a little or a lot of leakage. When quick changes in abdominal pressure occur, your muscles have to react quickly to make sure urine doesn't get pushed from your bladder. A cough or sneeze are great examples of a quick change of pressure in your body. Both are fast and forceful. If you have muscle weakness, there may not be enough strength to close the sphincters and stop urine from escaping (Diagram 3, Chapter 5).

Here is some background information to help you understand why there needs to be differences in the way you exercise these muscles in order for them to be effective for you. In every muscle throughout the body, there are fibers that react to slow movement (slow twitch) and other fibers that are fast twitch. Just like it sounds, the slow twitch are our endurance fibers. They can stay contracted for a long time and help to support our bodies and also work during standing, walking, or any activity that does not require quick or explosive motion. Conversely, the fast twitch fibers perform just as you would expect by working with the endurance fibers to add speed to the movement. These are the ones that kick in while running and, as you may have guessed, during that quick change in pressure to close off the sphincters and stop leakage.

The target for fixing stress UI is the fast twitch fiber. We want a very quick contraction before the pressure begins to increase to stop those drops from escaping.

If you are just starting, I suggest doing these exercises lying down with your legs propped up on pillows (hook-lying). It makes the exercises so much easier in the beginning because you are not working against gravity.

Make sure you feel a squeeze and lift before you move past Week 1. These are guidelines, if you feel you need to stay at a step longer, please do. It sometimes takes longer to perfect this exercise. Since it is crucial to program success, move through the steps only as you feel ready.

Stress Urinary Incontinence Exercise Program

Weeks 1-2 Kegel Program
- two-second hold to four-second rest
- ten times
- two times per day

Weeks 3-6 (Progress to sitting when able. Target at 4 weeks)
- two-second hold to four-second rest
- two sets of ten
- two times per day

and
- five-second hold to ten-second rest
- ten times
- two times per day

Week 7 and beyond (Progress to a combination of standing and sitting Kegels)

Add an additional set of ten repetitions to each of the above two and five second holds. At this point, you should be doing eighty to one hundred Kegels per day.

It is easier when you try to either schedule them throughout the day or fit them into your daily routine. For example, you could try doing some before you get out of bed, some sitting at lunch, or dinner. Some during commercials when watching television. And before you know it, you are done for the day! Space the exercises throughout the day so as not to tire the muscles –especially in the beginning.

Urge Urinary Incontinence Exercise Program

Urge UI, as you'll remember from Chapter 6, is having that strong sudden urge to urinate and leaking before you get to the toilet. It can be enough to wet your clothing. Urge urinary incontinence can also be accompanied by frequency, which again you will recall is going to the bathroom several times during the day. The program for this type of leakage addresses both leakage and frequency. For now, we will focus on the strengthening section and later in the chapter discuss frequency separately.

You will approach this strengthening program differently. You are going to work the muscle fibers that can hold a contraction longer. When the urge comes, the sphincter needs to close and stay closed until you either get to the bathroom or the urge passes.

Week 1-2 Kegel Strengthening Program (hook-lying)

- five-second holds to ten-second rest
- ten times
- two times per day

Weeks 3-6 (Progress to sitting. Target 4 weeks)

- five-second holds to ten-second rest
- twenty times
- two times per day

and

- ten-second holds to ten second rest
- ten times
- two times per day

Week 7 and beyond (Progress to a combination of sitting and standing)

Add an additional set of ten repetitions to each of the above five and ten second holds. At this point, you should be doing eighty to one hundred Kegels per day. These longer holds can be challenging to start. It is especially important to start the longer contractions in the hook-lying position. Progress as you become stronger.

Mixed Urinary Incontinence

Mixed urinary incontinence is two or more types of leakage, usually both stress and urge but not always. If you can't control bladder leaks when you feel a strong urge or have leakage during stress (cough/sneeze), you fit into this category, and you have a little more work to do. The Stress and Urge programs are combined to work on strengthening everything to combat your leakage.

The Mixed Urinary Incontinence Exercise Program

Make sure you can feel a lift and squeeze before you begin your program. Remember to start in hook-lying and progress when you are comfortable.

Weeks 1 and 2 Kegel Strengthening Program
- five-second hold to ten second rest
- ten repetitions
- two times per day

Weeks 3 to 6 (Progress to sitting. Target week 4)
- two-second hold four-second rest
- ten repetitions
- two times per day

and

- five-second hold and ten-second rest
- ten repetitions
- one to two times per day

and

- ten-second hold and ten-second rest
- ten repetitions
- one to two times per day

Week 7 and Beyond (Done in a combination of sitting and standing)

Add an additional set of *ten repetitions* to the above two and five and ten-second holds. At this point, you should be doing at least 100 Kegels per day.

When you look at these programs doesn't it look like you will be spending your entire day lying down doing Kegels? Once you get into a routine, they go pretty quickly. The easiest way when starting out is to try and do them in bed in the morning and at night. Depending on your schedule, daytime Kegels lying down might not be an option. Also, you are not doing them lying down forever. It is usually less than a month, depending on how consistent you are with the exercise program.

Once you become stronger, you should begin to do them in the sitting position. Once these are easy, then you can progress to a combination of sitting and standing. At this point, they should be a lot more convenient to do and you can do them anywhere—waiting for the light to change while driving or during commercials if you watch television. Make it work for your schedule. Getting through the first part is the most challenging.

Frequency and Nocturia

The last of the programs you will learn about have some similarities, but the approach to fixing them is different. Both have to do with two issues we have yet to discuss.

Urge and the Brain-Bladder Connection

As you have learned, urge is the signal you feel that tells you it is time to go to the bathroom. You will feel the urge as your bladder expands and fills with urine. Urine is constantly dripping into the bladder. You may feel the urge to go when it is filling. If everything is working as it should, you can usually ignore the initial urges without any consequences. If you have strong muscles and control, you may be able to even ignore a strong urge until it is convenient to get to the bathroom.

Whenever you feel the urge to go, you do not have to act on it. Some women would be in the bathroom every thirty minutes if they acted on it each time. The bladder does not fill quickly because there needs to be time for the kidneys to filter fluid. As you will recall, normal bladder habits mean that there are at least three to four hours between bathroom trips. As one ages, the time between voids can be every two and half hours. This is still considered normal.

What happens when you go to the bathroom when your bladder isn't full? First, there is generally not a lot of urine to empty. When you are running to the bathroom frequently and just a small amount comes out, you can start to change how often you act on the urge you feel to go. It is possible to extend the time slowly to increase the amount of time between bathroom visits.

Let's explore this a little further. The brain and the bladder work together. As the bladder fills, it stretches. Once it stretches to a certain point, it sends a signal to the brain that it is time to relax the muscles so you can urinate easily. You will feel a strong urge to go at this time. If your muscles and bladder are working normally, you can just go when it is convenient. If you have weakness, incoordination, or anything that disrupts the normal cycle, leakage may occur.

While the bladder is steadily filling and stretching, you may still have the urge to go. It can feel like a warning, telling you that the time is coming soon and when you are ready you should go.

What would happen though if every time you felt the urge you acted on it? Let's say it has been less than two hours so the bladder is probably not full; however, you really think you should go. You keep doing this regularly until it becomes a habit. You have trained your brain that it is expected that the bladder will always empty before it is full. That becomes the expectation. This is what can lead to frequency or going to the bathroom frequently without having a full bladder. This is a person that has the urge to go to the bathroom every hour. She goes to the bathroom and just a little bit of urine comes out. The bladder learns that it does not have to stretch to full capacity before it is time to empty. The timing between bathroom trips gets shorter and shorter. This is how a typical person with frequency would present.

The way to treat frequency involves retraining your bladder. It can be done. Once you determine how often you go to the bathroom, your goal is to try and lengthen that time in fifteen-minute increments. For example, if you find that you go to the bathroom every one and a half hours, try to add an extra fifteen-minutes to that time.

Urge Deference

Try these tips to help:

Once you get the initial urge, try not to go to the bathroom. Remember that urge is just a signal that you will have to go; it doesn't mean you have to go right now.

Stop and try to distract yourself. You can try a few Kegels to disrupt the signal that you have to go now. If you still have a strong urge, start to walk towards a bathroom. Do not rush to the bathroom, but try to take your time.

These techniques will add time in between voids. When you can, for a few days, wait fifteen minutes before you void without leaking. Continue to add in time in the same fifteen-minute increments. Your goal is three hours. Don't get discouraged with this. There will be setbacks since you are training from a learned behavior. This technique does work, so don't try to rush through it if you want success.

Nocturia

As we defined earlier, nocturia is getting up to go to the bathroom two or more times per night with or without leakage. The techniques you use for frequency can also be used for nocturia. You want to try and extend the time you are asleep and not wake up to go to the bathroom. Using the urge techniques are more challenging at night because it is hard to find a distraction in the middle of the night.

Here are some things that can give you more success. Try to stop drinking after 8 p.m. —earlier if you go to bed before 10 p.m. Do light leg exercises in bed prior to sleep, such as ankle pumps, ankle rolls, or leg raises. This is also a good time to practice your Kegels. After exercising, lie down for a few more minutes before getting up to go to the bathroom. If you take any medication that makes you go to the bathroom, consider asking your doctor if you can take it during the day so that you can sleep longer. If this is not possible, you may have to get up more frequently, and that is fine if this is the case.

The connection between the brain and bladder is strong. Changing these habits takes time and patience but it is possible.

CHAPTER 9

IS THERE ANYTHING ELSE I SHOULD DO?

....

Bladder Irritants

Although strengthening is very important to reach your goal of decreasing bladder leakage, there is more that can be done to help you to be successful. There are some foods and liquids that can be irritating to the bladder. When these are consumed, it may stimulate the bladder to want to empty before it is full. The key is finding out if any of these foods apply to you. Hopefully you don't consume everything that is on the list. Once you decide which foods you think might be causing more leaks or trips to the bathroom, you can start to eliminate them from your diet for a few weeks and see if it helps.

A nice tool to use if you have time is your bladder diary. The first time you completed one was to get an idea of your symptoms and to figure out the program that will help you. I generally don't have a patient do it again, but in therapy, I am able to help you figure out what might be the culprit. You may be using this book for self-help, and if that is the case, it is easier to use a diary.

Use a modified diary only if you don't have any idea if a food is increasing your bladder symptoms. You only have to start recording your symptoms after you have eaten the food. Afterwards, record your bathroom patterns for the next eight hours. If you see leakage, increased urge to go to the bathroom, or frequent trips to the bathroom, you have found at least one of your irritants.

Here is a list of the most common bladder irritants:

Coffee (regular or decaf)

This deserves a section on its own. All of you diehard coffee drinkers can take a minute to let that sink in. Usually when I tell the coffee drinkers that their symptoms may improve if they give up coffee for a few weeks, they look at me as if I am crazy and that is just not going to happen. It takes a lot of convincing to get cooperation on this one, but when they do, and see improvement, they feel it was worth it.

Some other irritants are:

- Alcohol
- Tomato based and acidic products
- Tea (regular and decaf)
- Spicy foods
- Sodas
- Caffeine and artificial sweeteners
- Milk
- And another big one—chocolate!

This is only a partial list. Please remember that you don't have to give these things up forever. You just have to learn how your body reacts to them and act accordingly. It is important in the beginning to eliminate them for a short time period because we are working on your muscle strength and control. Once that is improved, you will be able to handle holding your urine and not leaking or running to the bathroom as much. Think "I can do this. It is not forever."

Let's return to learning how your body reacts to certain foods. Let's say you have strengthened your muscles and have more bladder control but really want to start drinking coffee or tea again. Both of these are irritants in that they can cause you to have to go to the bathroom more often (frequency).

Go ahead and drink them, just be aware that you may have to go to the bathroom, so don't get in the car for a two-hour drive! Make sure you have the time and there is a bathroom nearby.

Tea is my bladder irritant, but I love it and drink it every day. I just know after my morning cup of tea, I will go to the bathroom a little more frequently. I don't have leakage, so I am okay with that. It's the price I pay for something I love. If I have an early flight, though, I might just have to enjoy that tea when I land. I don't like airplane bathrooms!

Concentrated urine is another bladder irritant. It is very important to drink water. As you may remember we discussed how drinking enough fluids can be an invaluable tool to keep your urine diluted and to reduce bladder irritation.

Exercise Program

Besides doing your Kegels regularly, there are more exercises that are helpful in increasing the strength and stability of the pelvic floor. As with any exercise program, start slowly and make sure you have your physician's approval to start any of these exercises. If there is any pain, stop immediately and consult your physician. If you cannot do the recommended number of exercises, do only a few repetitions and build slowly until you can comfortably do the program.

These exercises are especially helpful if you have pelvic muscle weakness and are not sure if you are doing your Kegels correctly. They strengthen the nearby muscles and help to support the pelvic area. These exercises are great to do if when doing a Kegel, you can feel a squeeze of the muscles but not a lift. Performing these additional exercises on a regular basis will help to strengthen your pelvic region.

Do each set one to two times per day
One set is ten repetitions

Hip Adduction
- Sit up straight in a chair with your feet on the floor
- Place a rolled towel or small ball between your thighs, close to your knees
- Squeeze your knees together for ten seconds and release
- Do one set per session
- Be sure your feet do not roll inward
- You should feel your inner thigh muscles working

Hip Abduction
- Tie an elastic exercise band around your knees in sitting position

- Separate your feet to hip width
- Press against the band separating your knees with your feet firmly planted on the floor
- Hold for ten seconds and release
- Do one set per session
- You should feel your outer thigh muscles working

Bridges
- Lie on your back on a flat surface
- Bend your knees and place your feet flat on the floor
- Keep your arms down at your sides
- Slowly lift your hips off the floor or bed as high as you can. Then, slowly lower
- Do one set per session

If you have any back problems or pain while doing this exercise, consult your doctor. Remember, none of these exercises should cause pain. If they do, you should stop immediately. When you are comfortable, add a Kegel while you are doing your bridges.

Diaphragmatic Breathing
- Start by sitting or lying down comfortably

- If you are sitting, make sure both feet are on the floor and you are sitting without slouching
- To make sure you are using the correct muscles and not chest breathing, it may be helpful to place one hand on your chest and one hand below your ribcage. If you are correctly using your diaphragm to breathe, the hand on your chest should remain still; only the one on your abdomen should move.
- Slowly inhale through your nose. You want to feel your rib cage open and expand as your belly rises.
- Slowly exhale through your mouth. You want to feel your rib cage close and come together. The abdomen should relax as your belly button lowers.
- If you are having trouble, make sure you continue to practice with your hand on your stomach to feel the rise and fall of your abdomen.
- Do five repetitions two to three times throughout the day.

Once you are comfortable, it would be beneficial to focus on relaxation through the pelvic floor to prepare your muscles for the work ahead.

Constipation

Long-term constipation can also be a contributor to weakening the pelvic floor. Constant straining and pushing can make the muscles too tight or too loose. Either situation can make it more difficult for the pelvic floor muscles to contract well enough to provide leakage control. Additionally, bearing down on the pelvic floor structures can cause them to shift downward resulting in pelvic organ prolapse. Pelvic organ prolapse happens when the muscles and ligaments that support the uterus, bladder, or rectum become weak or loose. Once this occurs the pelvic organs can drop or press into the vagina. If you suffer from constipation make sure you stay well hydrated and are eating enough fiber rich foods. Your physician will also be able to give you additional information to help. It is very important to do whatever is needed to reduce and eliminate constipation and straining as it can affect the health of your entire pelvic floor.

Modifiable Risk Factors

There is still more that can be done to help! Modifiable risk factors can be changed. For example; if you smoke or drink alcohol to excess, you can try to stop. Below are some risk factors that can contribute to weakening muscles and leakage:

- Smoking
- Excess weight
- Chronic constipation
- Excessive alcohol consumption
- Poor hydration
- Consuming bladder irritating foods
- Non-modifiable Risk Factors

Non-modifiable risk factors cannot be changed. These can include:

- Age
- Neurological disease
- POP or Pelvic Organ Prolapse
- Pelvic trauma
- Medications
- Decreased mobility

Having non-modifiable risk factors does not mean that there is nothing that can be done if you have leakage. For example, as one ages, the chances of experiencing some leakage increases for several factors. Post-menopausal women can have an increased chance of leakage. As estrogen in the body decreases, the bladder and urethra can weaken. In many cases, treatment can reduce or stop leaks.

There are also times when you need to seek professional help. If you have pain in your pelvis or abdomen, you should seek medical advice. Doing any of the exercises in this program should not cause any pain. If pain occurs, you should not continue until you have consulted with your physician or physical therapist. If you are diligent in the exercises and modifications and have not seen any improvement, there may be additional factors in play. Speak to your physician who may refer you to a specialist. There are several referrals that can help you. These can include:

- Urology
- Urogynecology
- Gynecologist
- Pelvic physical therapist

Don't give up! They may be able to identify the missing piece as to why you have not progressed. Once that is found, you can still be on your way to success with this program.

CHAPTER 10

HOW DO I KEEP MY PROGRESS?

....

Persistence

I have found that one of the greatest predictors of success with this program is understanding. Once you grasp the purpose of the pelvic floor and associated muscles, you can perhaps begin to see why leakage occurs. Another predictor will be your dedication to the program. It may seem overwhelming to follow this program to the end, but it can be done if you take it one step at a time and add in the next steps once you are comfortable. Your leakage did not happen overnight. It takes a while for the muscles to weaken enough to affect bladder control. Even in the therapy setting, it can take up to a month before you feel any difference in symptoms, and it is usually a small difference. Since you are doing this with the assistance of this book, it could take longer. If that is the case, don't get discouraged. You are on the right track if you are persistent in following the program.

Understand the Basics

You have identified your type of leakage and your Kegel program. You have practiced doing a Kegel and hopefully understand what you should feel. Once this step is mastered, you are well on your way to success.

Progression of Kegels

You have identified how to begin your program. As you get stronger, the exercises get easier to do. You have been doing your daily Kegel program. You started the program in the gravity eliminated position of lying on your back with your knees on pillows (hook-lying). This is the easiest position and can help you to master doing the contraction when you are not strong. The optimal progression in positioning is as follows:

Recumbent

We did not talk about this position earlier in the book; however, it is a good extra transition step if you are having difficulty moving from hook-lying exercises straight to sitting.

The recumbent posture is sort of a combination of both. In this position you are sitting with your upper body supported with pillows so that you are sitting up at around a forty-five-degree angle or higher. Your legs should be raised with a few pillows under your lower legs for comfort.

Sitting

Once you can confidently perform your exercises sitting, it becomes more convenient to do the exercises throughout the day. You can add them in when you are waiting at a red light or while watching television during commercial breaks.

Standing

Standing Kegels are difficult! It may be hard to feel a muscle lift in this position, however, once you are able to do a strong pelvic floor muscle contraction in sitting position, it is time to try some standing.

You want to master a good Kegel in a functional position. That is usually sitting or standing. Most of us are not able to spend our day lying down. This is a good practice posture, but it is not practical for the goal of stopping leakage. You will also want to increase the number of Kegels you are doing throughout the day. Remember, you are doing different hold combinations depending on your type of leakage:

- two-second holds to four-second rest
- five-second holds to ten-second rest
- Ten-second holds to ten-second rest

Don't try and do them all in one sitting. These are small muscle groups and can fatigue easily. You will want to space the exercises out throughout the day. Once your symptoms are better, you can reduce the number of repetitions per day as needed to remain dry and also maintain your strength.

Additional Exercise Program

The hip and core exercises you added with your Kegel program can still be done on a daily basis until your leakage has gotten better. Once you feel you have control, these exercises can be substituted for any exercises you normally did for hip and abdominal strengthening. You must remember that any exercise you do should first be cleared through your physician. Secondly, never hold your breath while doing these or any exercise. Increasing intra-abdominal pressure can be detrimental to pelvic floor health.

Regarding intra-abdominal pressure, if you have issues with constipation, please do whatever you can to improve your bowel health. The constant bearing down to eliminate can wreak havoc on your pelvic support muscles.

Pelvic Bracing

The pelvic brace is basically tightening the muscles in and around your pelvis and abdominal core to "brace" them for any change in posture or pressure. The easiest way to do pelvic bracing is by doing the Kegel exercise and slightly bringing your belly button towards your spine. You should feel your entire core and pelvic area tighten.

Practice pelvic bracing, and once you are comfortable, do a pelvic brace every time you:

- Cough
- Sneeze
- Lift a heavy object
- Walk up and down stairs

With regular practice and time, you should begin to remember to brace every time. Your goal is to do a pelvic brace every time until it becomes almost second nature and you automatically start to brace before you cough/sneeze, et cetera.

What to Do If Symptoms Return

Symptoms may return if you do not continue with some form of the program. Once you master the steps, the best practice is to make this is a lifelong habit. This does not mean you will be doing one hundred Kegels daily for the rest of your life. It does mean that there should be some Kegels done on a weekly basis. You can determine what your magic number is to maintain your progress.

If symptoms return suddenly, you should probably consult a physician; it may be a sign of something that needs to be medically addressed. If you begin to notice a slow regression, it is time to take action. Go back and refer to the steps in this book to see what you may need to add or go back to. When you had your first success, there may have been something that you did, in particular, that you really felt helped your symptoms. If you noticed something, go back and try that first. If you had success by reducing or eliminating leakage you can retrace your steps and again be successful. If your problem was urgency and you feel those symptoms returning, don't forget about your urge deference techniques. Be sure to pay attention to your body. Take action at the first sign of regression. This will be the most effective and least time-consuming way to keep moving in the right direction. It took a lot of effort to solve your problem, so let's make sure you remain successful and happy with the progress that you have made.

CHAPTER 11
CAN I REALLY DO THIS?

···

The answer is a resounding, yes! You can do this. Just remember it will take time and it will take effort.

The majority of the patients that I have treated waited years before they sought treatment. A few chapters ago we discussed how easy it is to be in denial about bladder leaks. It is an uncomfortable and sometimes embarrassing topic for some. Sometimes leakage will come and go depending on certain circumstances; for example, illness, medications, or pregnancy. Other times it will start slowly, just a few drops here and there, until the leakage becomes bothersome. This is the point that many consider seeking help. I hope that this book has helped you to recognize the signs early and start to address them. Bladder leakage is not normal, and it is not a normal part of the aging process.

Over the previous chapters, we have outlined the steps you can take to decrease your leakage. It may seem overwhelming at first, but if you take it one step at a time, it is definitely doable. You have taken the first step, which is recognizing that leakage and going to the bathroom frequently is not normal. More importantly, you have also learned that incontinence can be reduced or eliminated. Treatment for incontinence has a high success rate. Following the steps in this book will help you a lot. Some of you may still need a health professional to help you on your journey. Sometimes Kegels can be really difficult to master for some; others can get it easier. When you start your program by using the information in this book or going to a pelvic health therapist, learning how to do a Kegel is what will take the most time. Once you are able to find the correct muscles to contract and strengthen, you are on your way to progressing and seeing results.

Even if you do need to see a pelvic health PT, you will still have an advantage since you know what to expect and the general basis of the program. You can be more proactive about your treatment since you have some background knowledge. This is always a plus for you and the treating professional. We love clients that take initiative with their own health! I would be remiss if I didn't remind you that every therapist or physician has their own way and method of treatment. Even if their program differs somewhat, some aspects of the treatment process will be similar.

Take a minute to remember what your life was like before you ever had to think about your bladder leaks. Now, place your intention that you want to go back to that feeling and not have to worry about leakage again. I hope it has not been so long that you can't remember what it was like.

What If:

- You never had to remember which store had the best bathroom or even where the bathrooms are located in each store, restaurant, travel or rest center?
- You could enjoy a movie without interruption?
- You could laugh as hard as you wish and not worry?
- You could go out and not be anxious about leaking?

Those times don't have to be a wish, you can make them a reality!

Bladder leaks can sneak up on all of us. We are all busy. We begin to make the small adjustments that we need to accommodate the few drops that begin to escape on occasion. Maybe it's wearing a pantiliner, so you are not inconvenienced during the day. Then one day, you realize you have slowly made a lot of adjustments to deal with leakage. What was once a small change has turned into an entire lifestyle adjustment, and it happened so slowly you didn't see it coming.

There was a time when you were not even thinking about leakage. I want you to go back to that time and ask yourself: what would I give not to have this problem? What value would it have for you to try and live a better life? If you are ready to go back to a time when leakage was not even a thought, then you are ready to work on the solution.

The main thing this program will take for you to see results is time and effort. If you are motivated for a change, then know this is something you can do. You will need to do some exercises daily and really focus on perfecting your pelvic floor muscle strengthening. Don't let that stop you. You have all the information you need to start your strengthening program. Almost everyone I have treated has a similar concern, which is, *when will I have the time to do all of this?* As we move step-by-step through the program, you will begin to realize that you do have the time. Of course, once you begin to see results, you will also have the motivation to continue.

The exercises do not take as long as you think. If you don't believe me, go back and add up the number of repetitions of each exercise and how long you need to hold the muscle contraction for pelvic floor strengthening. For stress urinary incontinence, it is only two seconds! The muscle holds for urge incontinence are, at most, ten seconds. The most effective way to ensure success is to find a time and schedule that works for you and then schedule it. Look at it as an appointment. Once you get into a routine it will help tremendously with consistency. As you progress through the program it gets easier, especially when your Kegels can be done sitting or standing. They can be added anytime during the day, so there is no excuse not to get these done daily. Be inventive. Even some of the additional exercises can be done on break at work or incorporated into any other exercise program you may be doing.

Take the time to consider what you would need to change in your daily schedule for this to work. Once your routine becomes familiar and you can do the exercises from memory, try to set aside twenty minutes, twice per day. That seems like a small amount of time for peace of mind, less worry, and less stress.

Let's go back to our original question at the beginning of this chapter. Do you think you can do this? I sincerely hope that your answer is still *yes*. You know what needs to be done. Go at your own pace, stay consistent, and you will see the results that you desire.

CHAPTER 12

MAKE YOUR SUCCESS PERMANENT

....

Ann Marie came to therapy afraid and worried that she will always have to wear a pad and even progress to adult diapers for her bladder leaks. Even when wearing a pad, she was fearful that one day she would leak through her clothes, especially when she was out with friends or, even worse, at work. She had leakage for years; first starting as a few drops but now it is every day. Although it was an inconvenience, it was manageable as long as she used a bladder-leak pad. Following her annual doctor's visit, she confided that she was concerned about not being able to control leakage. Fortunately, her physician suggested she try pelvic physical therapy and she was placed on my schedule.

During our first visit, she let me know that she did not have a lot of confidence that this would work. Like many people, she had never heard of pelvic physical therapy. We spent a lot of time during this visit discussing my experience and the success that I have had previously working with patients that had her same problem. Her concern was that she did not think she could be helped. Incontinence has a great success rate! Research supports this. We talked about how improving her leakage could improve her life by reducing her fear of leakage in public. I was able to convince her to try the program for six weeks, as it may take that long to start to see improvement. She had leakage for several years, and since it was long-term, I told her it may take longer to see results. By that time, her leakage should be less, and if she did not see improvement, we could re-evaluate what she needs to change, she could return to her doctor, or both. She had to promise me, though, that during the six weeks, she had to work consistently. She finally agreed as she was so frustrated with her current leakage problem.

Findings during the internal part of the evaluation included poor pelvic muscle strength. There was no pain or muscle tightness, making her a great candidate for achieving improvement of her symptoms. Poor muscle strength is a common reason for urinary leakage. We followed the same program that you have access to in this book. We started by identifying her type of leakage using her symptoms recorded in her bladder diary. The next step was to start learning how to strengthen her pelvic floor muscles. It took a lot of practice, but she was able to learn how to do an effective Kegel. Once she was able to strengthen the correct muscles, she added the other exercises that we learned in chapter 9. Additional changes were incorporated throughout the program, which included reducing her coffee consumption, as that was her bladder irritant.

Ann Marie was very diligent in doing the program since she was so tired of living with the fear of a bladder leak in public. She got into the routine of doing her exercises daily, some at her desk for ten minutes, ten to fifteen minutes at night, and also practicing Kegels whenever she was stopped at red lights while driving.

The hardest step was the first one—making the decision to work on the problem. Once she made the decision, we were ready to go!

Ann Marie began to see improvement, and her entire attitude changed; she began to believe and have hope that she could manage her leakage. Each week there was improvement; she noticed less leakage, and one day she realized her pad was dry. There were no leaks that day! She continued to have less leakage, more dry days, and finally her leakage was under control.

During our last conversation she expressed that she wished more women knew that there is help. I hope that this book will be a resource and help another person learn that leakage is not normal. I believe, just like Ann Marie, you can follow this program and reduce, and hopefully eliminate, your leakage as well.

You are now able to recognize the signs and symptoms of urinary incontinence and hopefully see how it is affecting your quality of life.

In this book you have learned:

- How the bladder works
- What pelvic floor muscles are and their role in keeping you dry
- How to correctly perform a Kegel and strengthen your muscles
- What else you should do to be successful
- Different types of incontinence and what they mean
- The meaning of Stress UI
- The meaning of Urge UI
- The meaning of Mixed UI
- The meaning of frequency and nocturia.

How to Maintain the Progress You Make

You can do this! Just commit to a few months. For some of you, it may be faster, and for others a little slower, but you should notice some improvement. Remember, there may be some of you that need more help. If you have done the program with no improvement, you may need to see your gynecologist, urogynecologist, or pelvic physical therapist for additional help. That is okay. I want you to know that there is still hope that your leakage will be helped, but there may be another problem that needs hands-on help to identify first. If you need additional help and for specific questions, I can be contacted at: thepelvicdpt@gmail.com.

I hope many of you will be able to follow the program in this book and stop your bladder leaks. I wish that you can be free of worry of whether you will leak in public or be able to enjoy time with family and friends without interruption. I would love for your story to end like Ann Marie's at the beginning of this chapter. It is more than possible.

ACKNOWLEDGMENTS

....

Thank you to Angela Lauria and The Author Incubator's team, as well as to David Hancock and the Morgan James Publishing team for helping me bring this book to print.

THANK YOU

∙∙

I hope *To Pee or Not to Pee?* has given you a better understanding of how very common bladder leakage is and how it can be helped with the right program. You now have the tools and steps that can help you reduce and/or stop your leakage.

Stay consistent with the steps outlined. It may be challenging, but it will be worth working for to become leak free. It takes time to gain control of bladder leakage, so don't give up!

To improve your success, I would like to offer you a thirty-minute class to help get started. If you are interested in this offer, please email me at thepelvicdpt@gmail.com, so I can send you a link to access your free class.

Thank you to all of my past patients who encouraged me to write *To Pee or Not to Pee?* I would also like to thank each of you for supporting me by reading this book and doing the program. I wish you success!

ABOUT THE AUTHOR

· ·

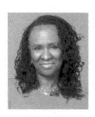 Dr. Shelia Craig Whiteman PT, DPT, CLT-LANA is a Doctor of Physical Therapy who specializes in pelvic health. She has successfully treated and helped hundreds of women reduce and eliminate bladder leaks. In addition to pelvic health physical therapy, Dr. Craig Whiteman is also certified in lymphedema and oncology rehabilitation.

She received a B.S. degree from Ithaca College and a Doctorate in Physical Therapy from Boston University. She is a licensed Physical Therapist in Maryland.

In addition to physical therapy and writing, Dr. Craig Whiteman is the owner of Interim Healthcare of Prince George's County, a home care agency which provides in-home services to seniors. As an advocate for health and wellbeing, she has led many presentations, fitness programs, and volunteer activities in her community. In her leisure time, she can be found teaching cycling and Pilates classes.

Certifications

Certified Lymphedema Therapist-CLT

Pelvic Health Therapist

STAR Oncology Clinician

Pilates Mat and Equipment Certification, PEAK Pilates

Certified Senior Advisor, CSA

Former member of Lymphology Association of North America, LANA

Contact email: thepelvicdpt@gmail.com.

9 781631 950742